Rose's Wellness

HEALTHY EATING COOKBOOK

KEEPING IT CLEAN
FOR HEALTHY WEIGHT LOSS & PREVENTATIVE HEALTH
GUILT FREE

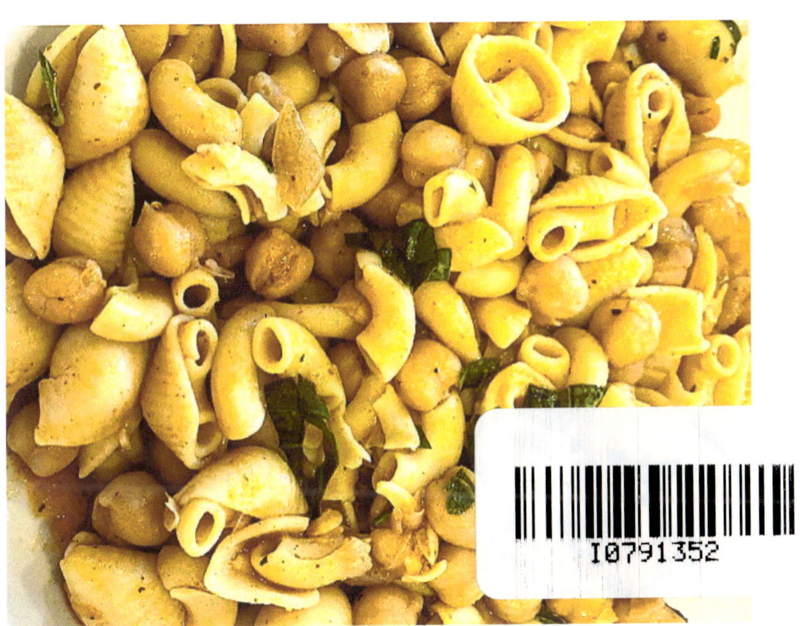

LOW GLYCEMIC

COMPLEX CARBS
SATISFYING
BALANCE

GUT FRIENDLY

NATURALLY GLUTEN FREE
COMFORTING
RELIEF

HEART HEALTHY

ANTI-INFLAMMATORY
HEALTHY FATS
FAT BURNING

By Rose Serluca

Table of Contents

Introduction- Learn how eating healthier and making better choices can help you achieve the results you want for healthy/sustainable weight loss and improved health. Simple & practical.

Testimonials- See from a few of my clients how a healthier lifestyle impacted their life, health & body.

Desserts- You can have your cake and eat it to, with out the guilt that is associated with dieting. Why, because it is a healthier version!

Breakfast- A healthy start to your day is a sure way to give your body the fuel it needs to keep you full and satisfied.

Dinners- A time to sit and feast on foods full of nutrients your body craves for balance & cell rejuvenation to turn your health around.

Smoothie- Easy to make smoothie, with simple ingredients.

Immune Booster Elixirs- Great way to help your body when your feeling down, fight illness or flu symptoms.

Bonus Grains List- Here is a food list of Low Glycemic/Naturally Gluten Free foods.

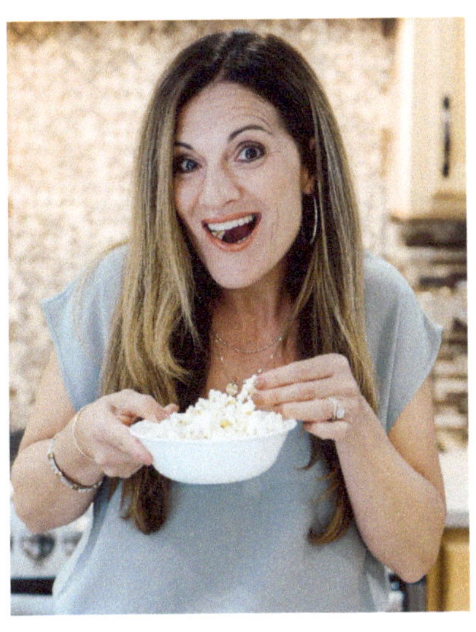

Food is key to a healthier lifestyle with out all the restrictions & struggles!

WELCOME TO A FEW OF MY FAVORITE RECIPES!

*INCLUDES 28 RECIPES,
Bonus Food List*

As a weight loss expert & an internal health specialist after seeing the miracles that have taken place within my clients' lives & health I've decided to share some recipes that I have used & created for my clients! I hope you enjoy these healthy recipes that can also help you target healthy weight loss, help prevent heart disease, balance blood sugars, improve gut health & more!
I dedicate this Ebook to my 3 sons Anthony (who has Type 1 Diabetes), Nico, Tommy & my husband Tommy. They have supported me, enjoyed these healthy recipes and allowed me to grow my passion which is to help people reach their health goals!
Rose Serluca~Rose's Wellness

Introduction-

Before you start to dive in... a message from Rose!
Are you struggling with weight loss? Are you concerned about a health issue?

If so, you are in the right place! I'm here to help you!
I offer simple, sustainable solutions with food. I use a non diet approach, rather a holistic approach where you get to eat all the foods you love!
Food is medicine. Food is healing. Food is the key solution. So let's try not to restrict so much and learn how to love and enjoy the foods you eat, with NO GUILT!
Food can heal on a cellular level to help turn your health around.
Start by eliminating sugar, refined carbs, unhealthy fats and proteins. Start incorporating low glycemic sugars, plant based/naturally gluten free carbs (complex carbs), legumes, vegetables, fruits, healthy fats (olive oil, avocado), nuts, seeds, fish, chicken... just to name a few!
Start here with these simple recipes. Keeping it clean for healthy weight loss & preventative health. All these recipes are low glycemic/low carb, gut friendly, anti-inflammatory, naturally gluten free & heart healthy!
Providing you balance, comfort & relief!

Here are some of my clients who have used these recipes!

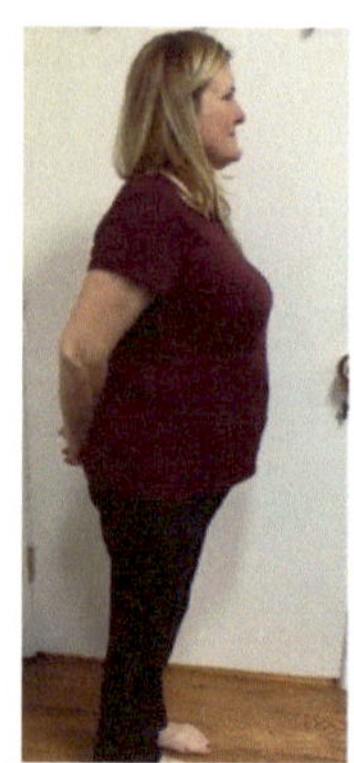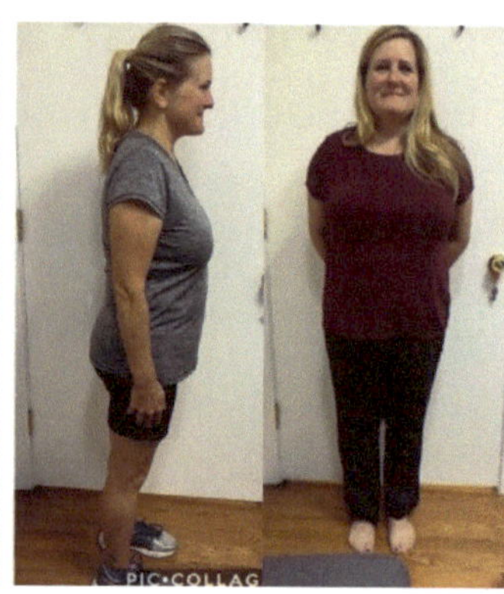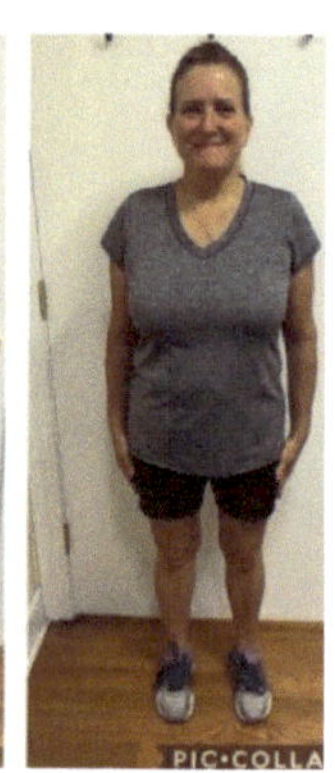

LOST 37 POUNDS
8 Week Course

"This has been a life changing experience for me and my husband. We both feel amazing and are making healthier decisions. My top 3 goals were to get gut healthy, reduce stomach pains that pertained to my diet, to stick to a healthy eating plan & lose weight to help reduce blood pressure & inflammation." "Rose has made this goal of mine possible and attainable!""Even my skin looks better!"

"I would recommend everyone I know to Rose, who is in need of change or has a health ailment they are suffering from!"

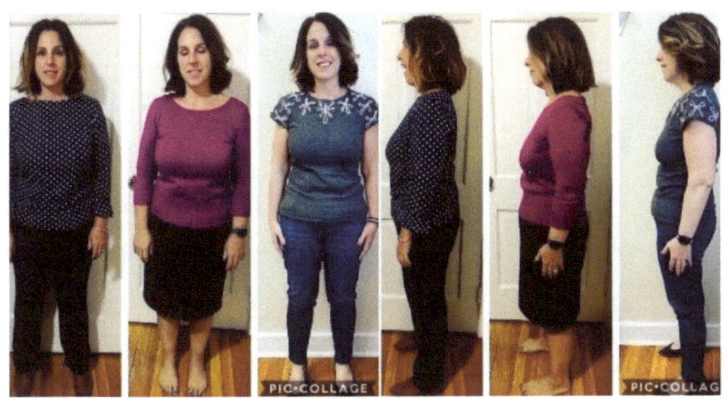

LOST 28 POUNDS
6 WEEK COURSE

What did you love about this?
"I loved the accountability aspect & learning healthier food choices. Because of this, I think about what I eat and don't just eat any food. I give it a little thought because good things happen now."
"I also love knowing how much to have of each food group. For example, eating more fish, eating low gluten & low sugar. I learned key aspects & gained a new lifestyle. I also learned which carbs to eat & WHEN to eat them."
"I cook super healthy, I prep the right foods with a lot of colors that make me feel good."

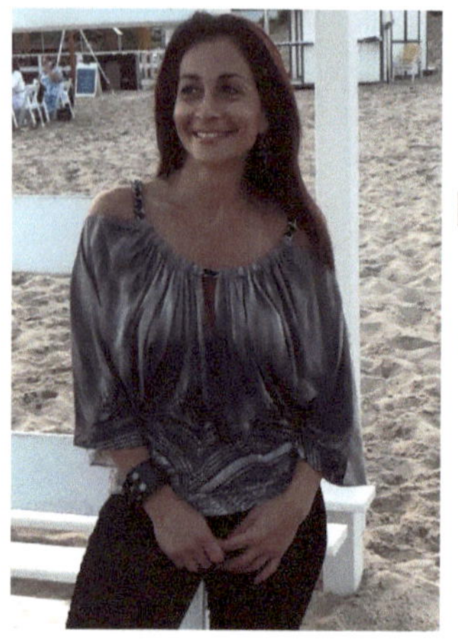

**LOST 4 POUNDS
IN 1 WEEK**

I can't thank Rose enough!
Her program was easy!
Before, I always stayed away from
carbs & now I eat them!
I lost my last stubborn 10 pounds!
My stomach issues are gone!
I eat more now, than when I was
on a my other diets!
This was real <u>simple with real
food.</u>

My cholesterol went down
100 points & triglycerides
down 385 points!
I battled dizziness &
nausea... <u>not anymore</u>!

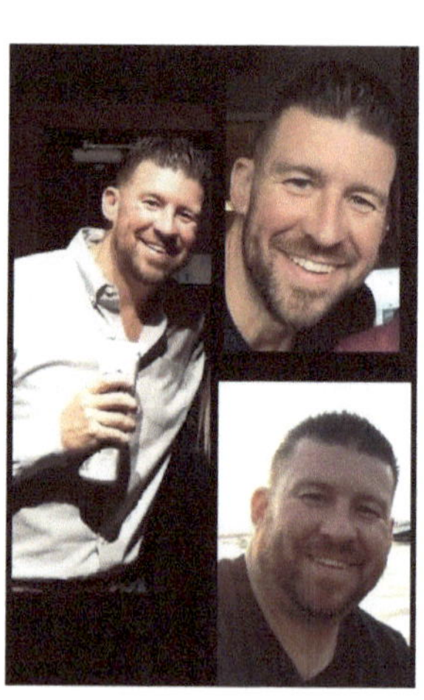

**LOST 60 POUNDS
IN UNDER 4
MONTHS**

Take note!
I've been in your shoes before!

I've tried every diet out there. I was just sick & tired of all the the guilt, the binging and the constant yo-yo dieting, until I stopped all this DIET MADNESS... I ended dieting & restricting, once & for all! That's when my life changed!

I've created the Life, Body & Health I've always desired!

Today, my mission is to do this for you as well!

Trust me, you don't have to give up the foods you love, instead just learn how to replace or swap them out with a healthier choice.

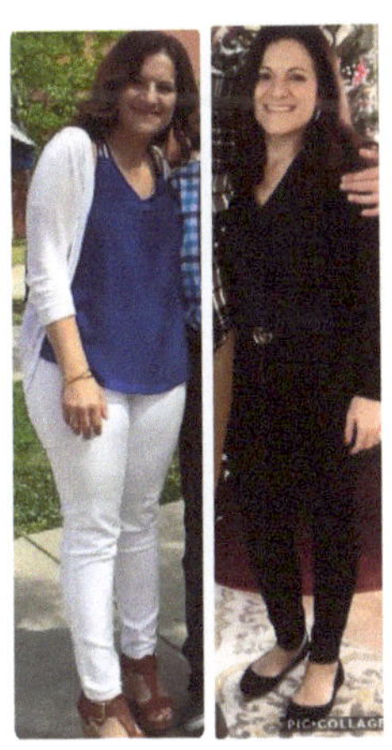

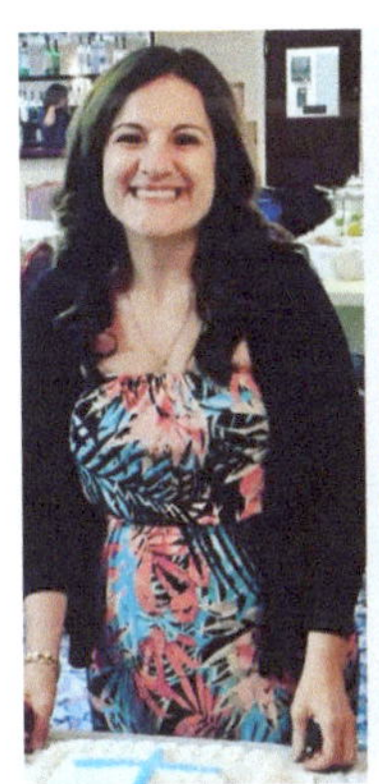

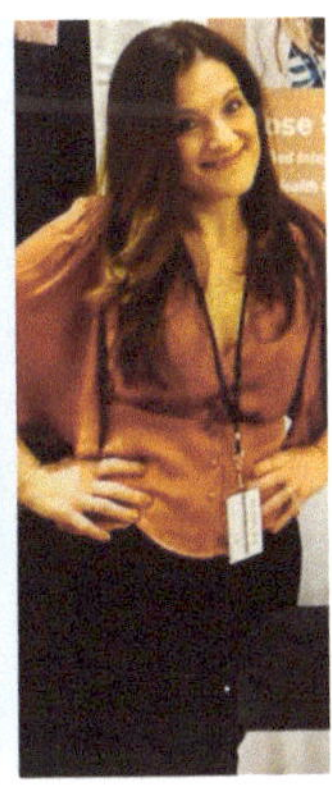

Let's start with dessert!

We all love dessert and we should enjoy desserts with no guilt! When you use naturally GF flours, healthy fats and low glycemic sugars... then why not! You have no reason not to!

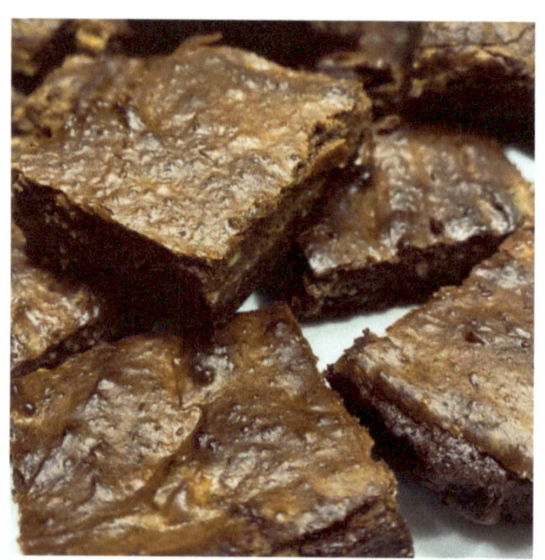

GF Brownie & Cheesecake Swirl

<u>Ingredients-</u>

<u>For the brownies:</u>
8 tablespoons butter (melted),
1/2 cup Coconut Sugar,
1/3 cup unsweetened cocoa powder,
2 eggs beaten,
1/4 teaspoon salt, 3/4 cup almond or oat flour

<u>For the cheesecake layer:</u>
4 ounces softened cream cheese,
3 tablespoons monk fruit,
2 tablespoons unsweetened almond milk,
2 teaspoons vanilla extract

<u>Instructions</u>
Preheat oven to 350 degrees. Line an 8x8 baking pan with parchment paper. In a mixing bowl combine the melted butter, coconut sugar, and cocoa powder until completely combined. Mix in the eggs, stir well. Add the almond flour and salt, stir well. Mixture will be thick. Spread the brownie mixture to all four corners of your baking pan, set aside. In a blender or food processor add the cream cheese, monk fruit, almond milk and vanilla extract and blend for 15 seconds, scrape down the edges and blend again. Spoon the cheesecake mixture in lumps onto the brownie batter, and swirl. Bake for 25-30 minutes or until brownies are set. Allow to cool and slice. Store in the refrigerator.

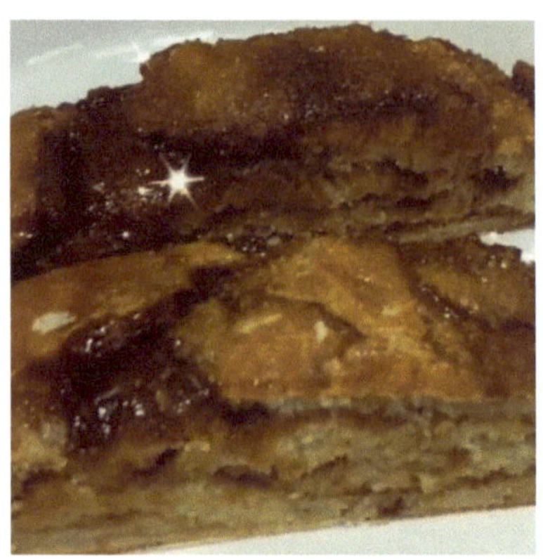

GF Cinnamon Roll

Ingredients-
For the Dough-
-2 large bananas
-1 1/2 Cup of all (1:1 GF, Almond, Oat,
I combined all 3) You may need more later,
if too watery after you use milk
-1 1/2 TBLS baking powder
-3-7 TBLS almond milk (Start with less at first)
For the Filling-
-4 TBLS coconut sugar
-1 1/2 TBLS cinnamon
*Melted Coconut oil or Ghee for brushing
For the Glaze-
-1-2 tsp of vanilla extract -2 TBLS of Ghee or Butter -2 oz
(roughly 1 TBLS) of Cream Cheese *Butter and Cr. Cheese
Softened* -1-3 TBLS of Almond Milk Depending on how
creamy you want it -3 cups of Confectionary Sugar *Add 1
cup of C. Sugar at a time when blending*

<u>Instructions-</u>
1. Mix all the dough ingredients together in a bowl until a dough forms, (I used a potato masher). Use a little almond milk at a time and only add as needed to keep it from getting too wet/sticky. If you add too much almond milk just add a little more flour until a thick dough forms (not too much or it will come out dry). Dough should be thick but may be a little sticky. 2. Roll out dough with hands on a floured surface, using your hands to press out like you would a pizza doe, but rectangular. (sprinkle flour on dough and hands to prevent sticking) Be sure not to make it too thin and doe should not be sticky at this point. 3.Brush with melted coconut oil or ghee. 4. Sprinkle the cinnamon sugar mixture on top and spread evenly. 5. Roll up dough. Cut in equal slices if you want to make buns or roll out to make a roll and cut later (that's what I did). 6. Bake on a cookie sheet and parchment paper for the roll at 350 for 20-25 minutes or use a glass pan greased or parchment paper and add cut out pieces and bake, may need extra time for baking because ovens vary.
<u>Icing Instructions-</u>
In a medium bowl and a hand held mixer add 1 cup of confectionary sugar, vanilla, softened butter and cream cheese and mix then add another cup of confectionary sugar and 1 TBLS of milk and repeat with one more cup of confectionary sugar and add more milk if necessary and how creamy you want it. Enjoy!

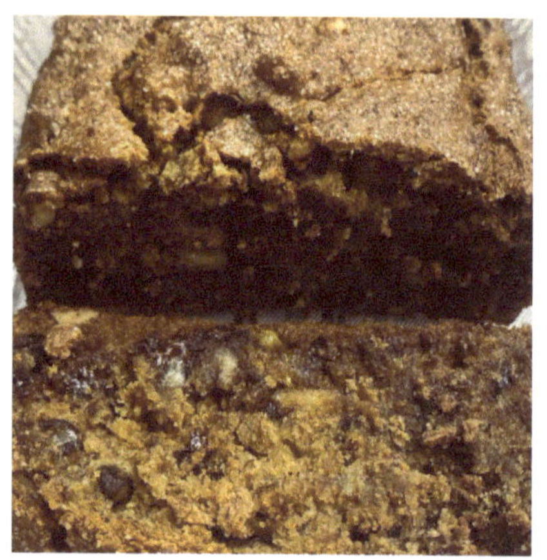

BEST GLUTEN FREE
BANANA BREAD

THIS IS THE BEST! IT'S EASY, MOIST & AN ALL IN ONE
BOWL RECIPE!
My kids & hubby said it's the best they've ever had!

<u>INGREDIENTS-</u>
3 ripe bananas (mashed),1/3 cup butter (melted),
3/4 cup coconut sugar, 1 egg, 1 teaspoon vanilla, 1&1/2
teaspoon baking soda, 1&1/2 teaspoon baking powder,
1/4 teaspoon cinnamon, 1 pinch teaspoon salt, 1&1/2
cups GF Flour (I used 1:1 flour and Almond Flour
combined), 1/2 cup chopped walnuts, 1/2 cup of
chocolate chips.

INSTRUCTIONS-
Preheat oven to 350 degrees F. Spray a loaf pan with baking spray. In a large bowl, combine the mashed bananas with the melted butter, then add the sugar, egg, and vanilla. Stir well with a large wooden spoon. Add the baking soda, baking powder, cinnamon, and salt and stir to combine all ingredients. Add the flour. After flour is mixed in add the walnuts & chocolate chips and stir it all up. Pour the batter into the greased or lined loaf pan. Bake for 50-60 minutes, until a tooth pic or knife inserted in the center of the loaf comes out clean.

Cool in the pan for 10 minutes, then turn it onto a plate long enough to cool completely.

Cut, serve & enjoy!

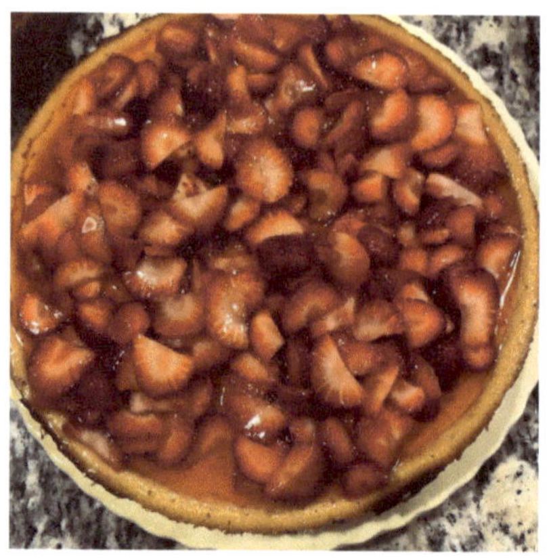

GF CHEESE CAKE

<u>INGREDIENTS</u>
<u>Crust-</u>
1 cup Almond or Oat Flour, 4 TBLS butter,
1 tsp cinnamon
<u>Cheesecake/Filling-</u>
(2) 16 oz cream cheese, 4 eggs, 2 tsp
vanilla extract, 2 tsp fresh lemon juice,
1 pinch salt, 1/2 cup sweeter (coconut
sugar or monk fruit). Refrigerate for at
least 5 hours to make firm.
<u>Toppings-</u>
2 TBLS of sliced strawberries, 1-2 TBLS
monk fruit. Mix all together & top before
serving!

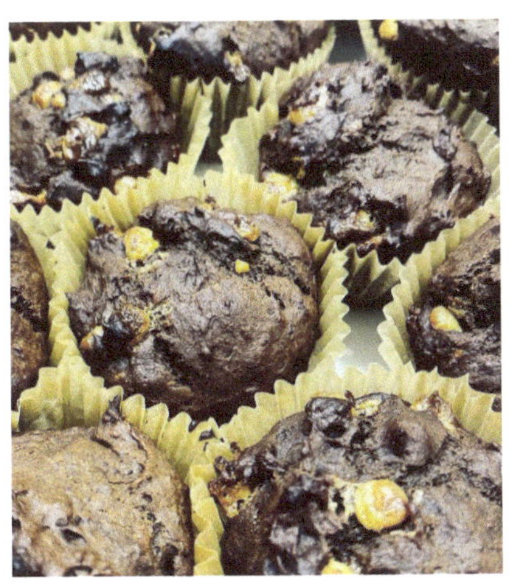

3 INGREDIENT GF MUFFINS

<u>INGREDIENTS-</u>
2 Ripe Bananas, 3 TBLS Creamy Unsweetened Nut Butter, 3 TBLS Unsweetened Cocoa
OPTIONAL- The mix-ins of your choice (chocolate chips, walnuts, coconut flakes, almond slices, etc.)
<u>INSTRUCTIONS-</u>
Preheat oven to 350 F. Use a food processor to combine all of the ingredients (except for your optional mix-ins) until well blended. Use a spatula or spoon to fold in a handful optional mix-ins.
Fill 6 cupcake liners evenly to the top. Bake for approximately 15 minutes.
Let cool, and enjoy!
They are sweet and taste like fudge!

FROZEN DARK CHOCOLATE BANANA POPS

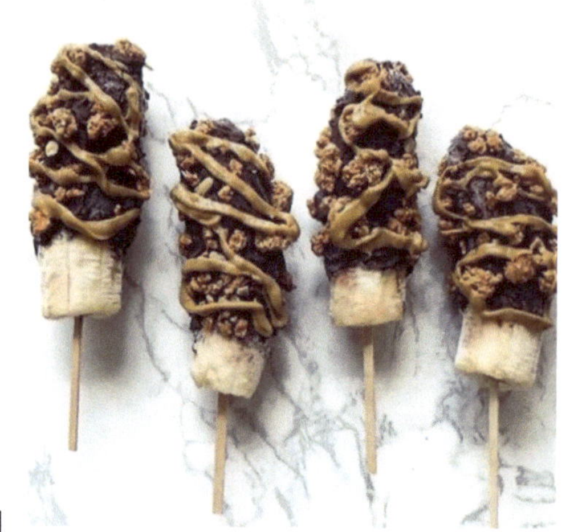

INGREDIENTS
-4 bananas, cut in half
-1/2 C cacao powder
 -1/3 C melted coconut oil
-1 tbsp agave
-Organic almond or nut butter of your choice with no added sugars
 -1 tbsp of any chopped nuts (walnut, almonds, pecans...)

INSTRUCTIONS
1. Peel & cut bananas in half. Then pierce with a wooden skewer or a popsicle stick.
2. To make the dark chocolate, combine Cacao powder, melted coconut oil, & agave in a medium bowl. Stir until smooth.
3. Dip bananas in chocolate. Roll the nuts before placing them on a baking sheet lined with parchment paper.
4. Drizzle with nut butter.
5. Store in the freezer & enjoying.
Makes 8 banana pops.

One Bowl Cakes

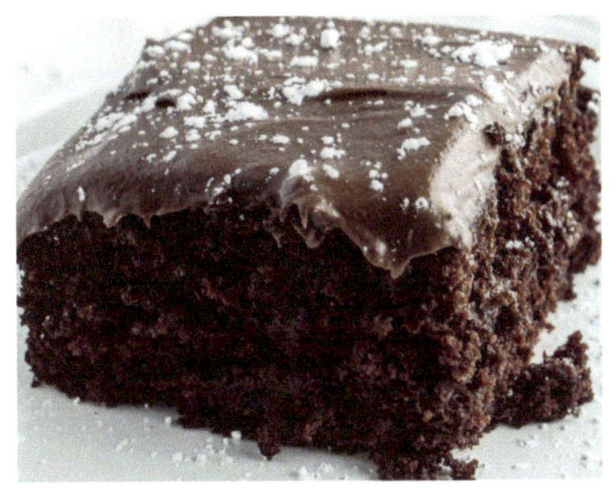

GF Chocolate Cake

<u>Ingredients-</u>
1 1/2 cups Almond
1:1 GF Flour or combined
1 cup coconut sugar
1/4 cup unsweetened cocoa powder
1 teaspoon baking soda
1/2 teaspoon salt, 1 cup cool water
6 Tablespoons canola or avocado oil
1 Tablespoon distilled white vinegar
1 teaspoon vanilla

<u>Directions-</u>
Preheat oven to 350° F. Grease or line with parchment paper a 9-inch round pan or a 8x8 pan.. Mix all dry ingredients into a bowl and set aside. In a measuring cup combine water, oil, vinegar, and vanilla. Add liquids to bowl & gently stir until there are no lumps (about 30 seconds). Pour into pan and bake for 30 minutes. Cool completely in the pan and frost, glaze, or dust with powdered sugar.

Lemon Cake

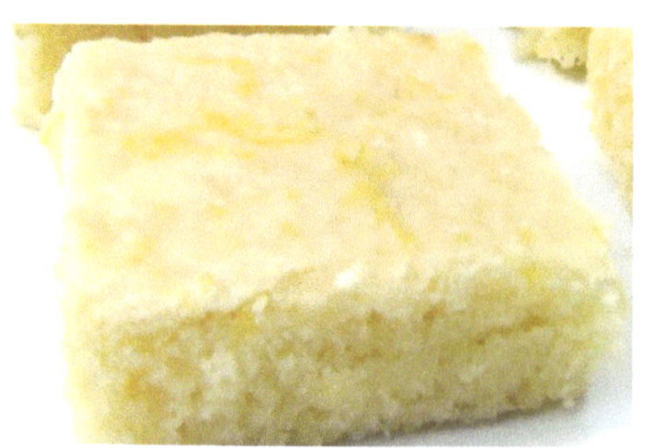

Ingredients-
1 cup 1:1 GF Flour, 3/4 cup monk fruit sugar
1/4 teaspoon salt, 1/4 teaspoon baking soda
2 eggs, 1/4 cup plain or vanilla Greek yogurt
3 Tablespoons avocado or canola oil
Grated zest of 2 lemons
2 Tablespoons fresh lemon juice

Glaze-
1 cup powdered, sugar zest of 1 lemon & about 2 to 4 Tablespoons fresh lemon juice

Instructions- Preheat oven to 350°. Line an 8 x 8 or 9 x 9-inch square pan with foil or parchment paper. Put all ingredients into a bowl. Stir by hand until smooth. Pour batter in pan and bake for about 20 minutes. Let cool in the pan for 10 minutes. Lift out of pan and spread glaze over the cake.
For the glaze- Stir glaze ingredients together in a bowl, adding juice gradually until glaze is spreadable.

Super Healthy Grab & Go
Banana Energy Cookies

Ingredients:

2 ripe, medium bananas, 1 cup rolled oats, 1/4 cup pumpkin seeds (or any seeds you like),
1/4 cup of coconut sugar, 1/4 cup shredded unsweetened coconut ,1/4 cup berries, 1 Tablespoon chia seeds, 1/2 teaspoon cinnamon , Pinch salt

Directions:

1. Preheat the oven to 350
2. Line a baking tray with parchment paper and set aside.
3. In a small bowl, mash the banana. Set aside.
4. Combine the rest of the ingredients in a large bowl.
5. Add the mashed banana to the dry ingredients & mix.
6. Let the mixture stand for five minutes to absorb the moisture from the banana.
7. Use 1/4 cup of the mixture and mold together to form a round cookie.
8. Place the cookie on the lined tray.
11. Bake for 15 - 20 minutes, or until the cookies are golden.
12. Remove from the oven, then transfer to a rack to cool completely.
13. Keep for up to two days in an airtight container, or freeze for later.

5-Ingredient Flourless Banana Chocolate Chunk Oatmeal Mini Muffins

<u>Ingredients</u>
3 medium ripe bananas, mashed, 2-1/2 cups old fashioned or quick cooking oats
1 teaspoon baking powder, 1 large egg
1 cup dark chocolate chunks or chocolate chips or unsweetened chocolate chips

<u>Instructions</u>
1. Preheat oven to 350°F. Spray a 24-cup mini muffin pan with non-stick cooking spray.
2. In a large mixing bowl, add the mashed banana, oats, baking powder and egg. Mix or stir until well combined. Stir in the chocolate chunks.
3. Scoop batter evenly among prepared mini muffin cups (filling up to 3/4).
Top each muffin with an additional chocolate chunk, if desired.
Bake for 12-14 minutes or until the muffin tops look set and oats are just starting to crisp on top.

Breakfast should be a great start to your day for energy!

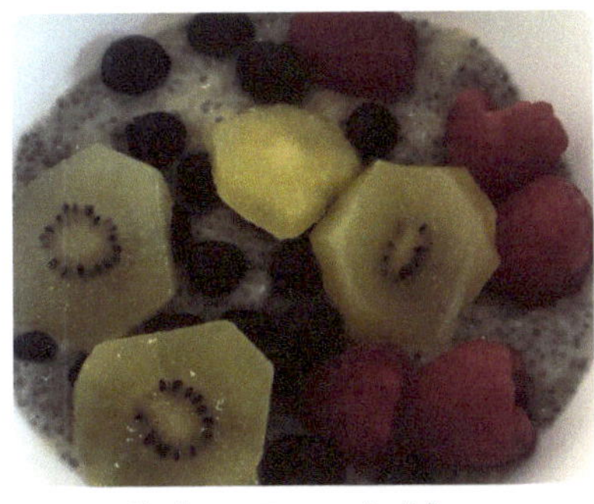

Chia Pudding

QUICK 3 INGREDIENT CHIA BREAKFAST-
1 Mashed Banana- 2 TBLS Chia Seeds
-1/3 C Unsweetened Nut Milk
Let sit in fridge for at least 15 min or overnight.
Top with Blueberries or your favorite fruit.

Simple, Just slice up a sweet potato and either bake it with salt and pepper or put in your toaster oven and cook till toasted then season after!
Top with your favorite toppings! Eggs & avocado or nut butter and banana...

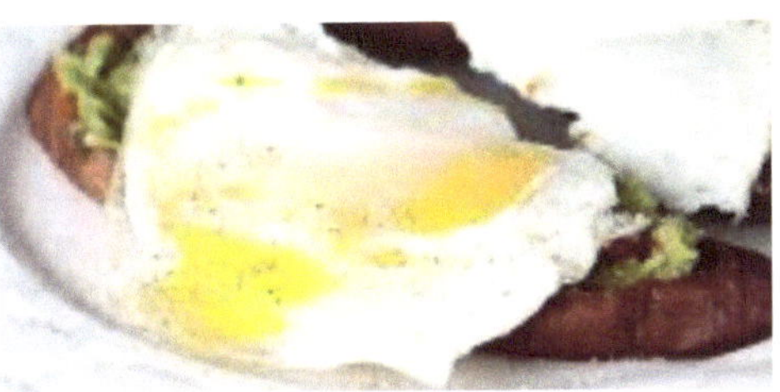

Sweet Potato Toast

Baked Avocado and Egg Recipe

<u>Ingredients-</u>

1 organic avocado, halved with pit removed, 1 egg, salt, pepper, your favorite seasoning

<u>Instructions-</u>

Directions- Preheat the oven to 425 degrees F.
Cut a little bit of the rounded bottom part of the avocado to help avoid spilling the egg. Place the avocados in a baking pan or a muffin pan to help it to stay in place. Whisk the egg in a bowl, divide it between the avocado holes. Sprinkle with salt, pepper and the seasoning. Bake for 16-18 minutes, until the egg has fully set.

Sweet Potato Toast With Toppings

<u>Ingredients-</u>

-1 small sweet potato sliced into (1&1/2 inch slices)
-1⁄2 avocado, mashed -1 teaspoon garlic powder
-1 teaspoon cumin -1⁄2 teaspoon Himalayan salt
-1⁄2 teaspoon black pepper (optional) -1⁄2 tomato, sliced
-1 teaspoon any seeds

<u>Directions-</u>

1. Place sweet potato slices in toaster until browned.
2. In a bowl, mash the avocado, garlic powder & spices.
3. Spread on sweet potato slices.
4. Place tomato on top mash & sprinkle with seeds.

Stuffed Pepper Breakfast Recipe

<u>Ingredients</u>
4 bell peppers, sliced in half, core and seeds removed
8 eggs, beaten, 1 cup sliced mushrooms,
1 diced onion, 3 cups baby spinach 1 tomato, diced
½ tsp. garlic powder, cooked bacon, ham, or sausages,
 (optional), 1 tbsp. olive oil, sea salt, black pepper

<u>Instructions-</u>
Preheat your oven to 375 F.
Use olive oil in a skillet placed over medium-heat.
Sauté the onion until soft, about 4 minutes, then add the
mushrooms and tomatoes and cook about 2 minutes. Add
the spinach and cook until wilted, about 1 or 2 minutes.
Season to taste with salt, pepper, and garlic powder.
Divide the vegetable mixture equally among the bell
pepper halves. Top off each bell pepper half with some of
the beaten eggs, and add the meat of your choice, if using.
Place the stuffed peppers in the oven on a baking sheet,
and bake for 40 minutes.

DINNER RECIPES

You can eat pasta! Why... Because here I use legume pasta which has many health benefits. It is low glycemic, has lots of fiber & protein that will satisfy you longer than your traditional white or wheat pasta that has no nutritional value that gives you NO ENERGY and stores fat instead! Eating this type of pasta will help you burn fat!

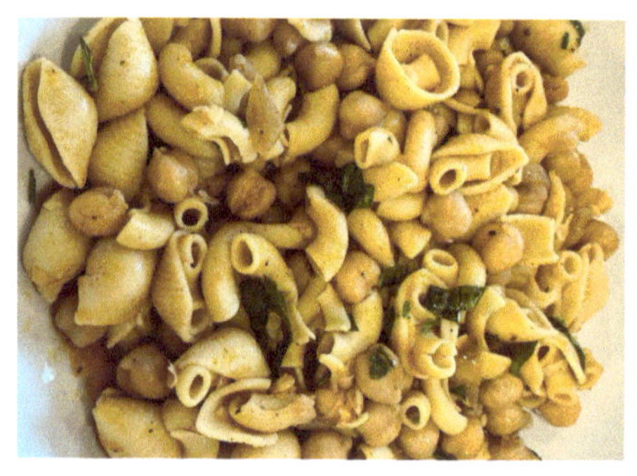

PASTA E CICI

<u>Ingredients</u>- 2 Cans of organic chickpeas
(rinse beans & fill with clean water, keeping beans in can)
-olive oil -1 chopped onion -4 minced garlic cloves -salt
-pepper -Italian seasoning -bay leaf -2 tsp of paprika
-1 pound of cooked red lentil or chickpea pasta
<u>Directions</u>- Sauté onion and garlic in olive oil and lightly cook. Add 2 cans of chickpeas with the water. Add all seasoning. Cook on medium heat for about 15 min with cover on. Add pasta and mix together. Add some chopped fresh basil & parsley- ENJOY!

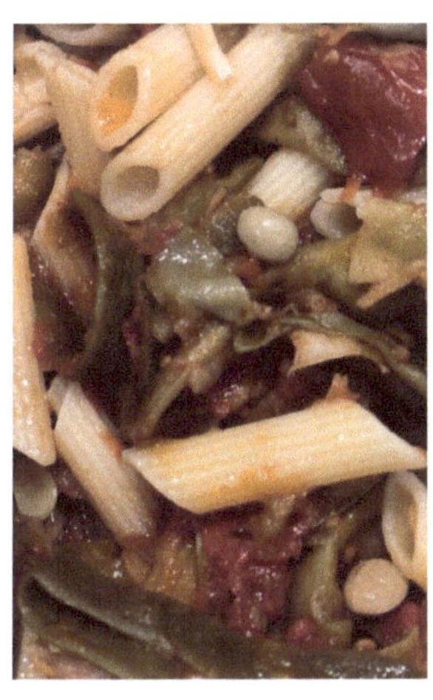

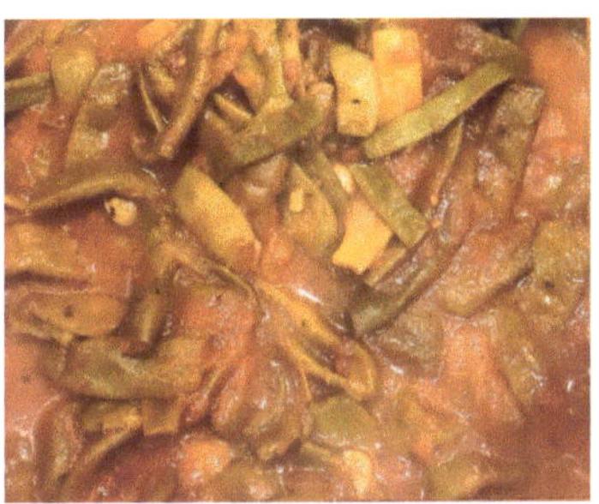

PASTA E FAGIOLI

So easy to make!
1. Sautee Garlic & onion in olive oil.
2. Add the Fagioli (Italian flat beans)
 (maybe 2-3lbs), if you don't have fresh use string beans.
3. Add fresh tomatoes (about 2 pounds) or 2 large cans of diced tomatoes and 1 small can of tomato paste if you want a thicker sauce & add a little water depending on how thick you want your sauce.
4. Add salt, black pepper, oregano, basil, parsley, & bay leaf!
5. Optional: add cooked legume pasta for healthier low carb/naturally GF dish!
6. Sprinkle some Romano or parmesan cheese. Mangia! Mangia!

You want to try to incorporate some lean protein that are anti-inflammatory, to help with chronic illnesses, autoimmune disorder, diabetes, high blood pressure, high cholesterol, obesity, etc...!

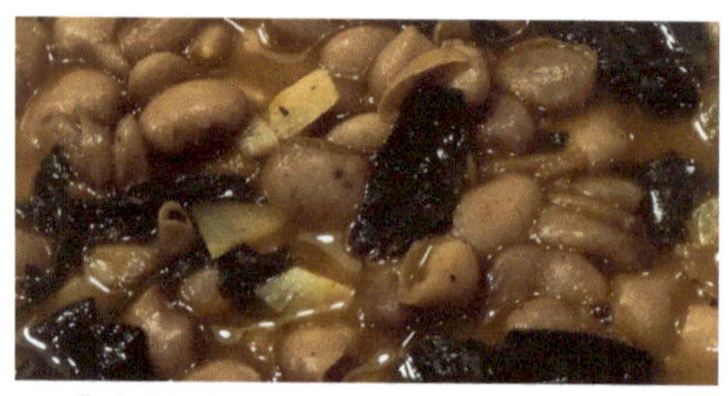

QUICK BEAN SOUP

<u>INGREDIENTS</u>
4 minced cloves garlic,
1 onion, olive oil,
2 cans of kidney or pinto beans,
1 bag of spinach or kale
salt, pepper, 1 TBLS of paprika
Italian seasoning & oregano.

<u>DIRECTIONS</u>
Sautee garlic & onion with olive oil in a medium sauce pan. Add 2 cans of the beans (rinsed & add back fresh water in can with the beans before pouring in the pan), add your leafy greens bag (cook down), add about 1-2 cups of water depending on how liquidy you like it, add seasonings. making sure you add at least 1 TBLS of paprika. Cook for atleast 15 minutes.

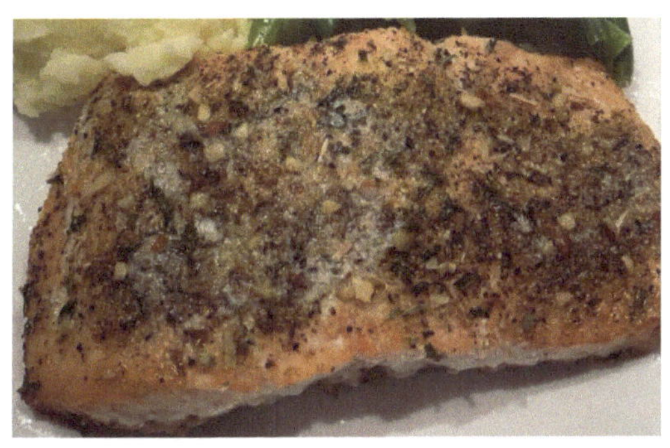

SALMONE DELIZIOSA

<u>Ingredients & Directions-</u>
Use 6-8 pieces of 4-8 ounces of salmon pieces
(leaving skin on)
In a bowl add melted coconut oil (1-2 TBLS),
juice of 2 lemons (set aside the lemons to slice
after & to place on top of salmon after all
ingredients are on top of salmon),
add salt, pepper, cilantro or oregano to the coconut oil &
lemon, mix all together and add on top of salmon, add
extra seasoning if you would like more flavor, add a sliver
of butter or ghee on each piece of salmon & place sliced
lemons on top for extra flavor!
Preheat oven to 425, bake on parchment paper or a
greased pan, uncovered for 20-30 minutes, depending on
how you prefer your salmon cooked- enjoy!! :)

Anti-Inflammatory Salmon Over Kale Salad

<u>Ingredients-</u>
-8 ounces of wild salmon, cut into two fillets (Skin on)
 -half a cup of parsley, chopped -half a cup of fresh basil chopped -one lemon juice -one garlic clove, chopped -1 teaspoon cayenne pepper -1 tablespoon nutritional yeast -2 tablespoons olive oil-1 teaspoon sea salt
-1 teaspoon black pepper -a quarter cup Pine nuts (optional) -four lemons slices

<u>Salad-</u>
3 cups kale, stems removed -3 tablespoons olive oil - 1lemon juice-1 teaspoon salt, 1 cucumber diced - 1/4 cup of Pepita seeds toasted -half a avocado diced

<u>Directions-</u>
Combine all the ingredients except for the salmon and lemon slices. Place the rest of ingredients in a food processor to form the greens mixture. Add more olive oil if it is too thick. Place salmon on a parchment lined baking tray. Top each fillet with greens mixture and place two lemon slices on each piece. Bake salmon in a preheated oven at 375° for approximately 20 minutes or until fish flakes. Place kale in a bowl and top with olive oil, lemon juice, and salt. Massage the kale leaves until tender and set aside for five minutes before adding cucumber, seeds, and avocado.

Chicken & Lime Recipe

<u>Ingredients</u>
2 lbs boneless, skinless chicken thighs or drumsticks,
4 tbsp olive oil, 4 minced garlic cloves,
4 tbsp. fresh cilantro or your favorite seasonings,
2 tbsp. lime juice, 1 tsp. red chili flakes, 1 tsp. cumin, salt & pepper.

<u>Directions</u>
In a bowl, whisk together all the ingredients, except for chicken.Add salt & pepper to taste.Add the chicken & let it marinate in the refrigerator, covered, for 1-2 hours. Preheat your oven to 375 F. Heat up some olive oil in a skillet and brown the chicken on both sides for 2 to 3 minutes. Transfer the skillet to the oven & bake for 15-20 minutes, or until the chicken is cooked through. Garnish the chicken with fresh seasoning and serve with lime wedges.

Chicken with Tomatoes & Asparagus

<u>Ingredients</u>
5 chicken breast or 10-12 drumsticks,
3/4 cup pitted olives, 1 diced bell pepper,
1 chopped onion, 1 bunch of trimmed asparagus,
 2 cups diced tomatoes, 4 minced garlic cloves,
1 1/2 cups tomato sauce, 1/4 cup chicken stock,
1 tsp. red pepper flakes,
1/4 cup fresh chopped parsley plus more to garnish
1/4 cup chopped fresh basil plus more to garnish, 2-4
tbsp. olive oil, salt & black pepper.

<u>Directions</u>
Season the chicken to taste with salt & pepper.
Use Olive Oil in a pan over medium-high heat; brown each
side of chicken 3 to 4 minutes. Remove the chicken & set
aside in a separate bowl. Lower heat and add more olive
oil to the skillet. Add the onion, bell pepper and garlic;
cook until soft. Add in chicken stock, bring to a simmer.
Add the asparagus, diced tomatoes and olives; cook for
about 5 minutes, then add in the tomato sauce. Sprinkle
the sauce with parsley, basil, red pepper flakes, and
season to taste. Toss everything and bring the chicken
back to the pan. Cover & cook until chicken is cooked.
Serve topped with fresh parsley and basil.

Calabrese Chicken

<u>Ingredients</u>
1 lb. chicken tenderloins, 1chopped onion,
3 minced garlic cloves,
12 oz. sliced mushrooms, 1⁄2 cup sliced sun-dried
tomatoes, 15 oz. can of diced tomatoes,
1 tsp. oregano, 1 tsp. basil, 1 tsp. parsley, olive oil,
salt and black pepper
<u>Directions</u>
    Use little olive oil in a large skillet placed over medium-high heat. Add the chicken and brown for 3 minutes on each side. Remove chicken and set aside on a plate.
Add some more oil to the skillet if needed. Add the sliced mushrooms in a single layer and brown for a few minutes per side. Remove from the pan and set aside.
Add the onion and cook until soft, about 4 minutes.
Add the garlic and sun-dried tomatoes and sauté for 2 to 3 minutes. Stir in the diced tomatoes and all the seasonings with salt and pepper to taste.
Transfer the chicken back to the pan.
Cover and cook until the chicken is cooked.
Return the mushrooms to the pan and mix it up. Add more seasonings if needed.

Sometimes we like a slice of bread... now you can!

Many times, my clients say... I miss a slice of bread now & then! The sliced sweet potato isn't cutting it for me when I want to have a slice with my eggs! LOL! I totally get it!

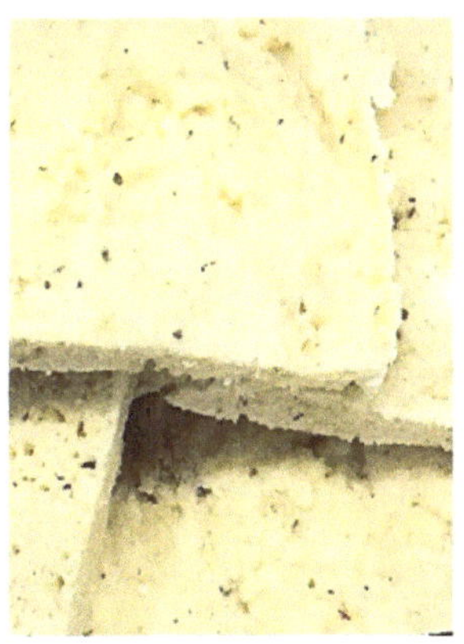

Keto Bread

For quick microwave 90 seconds!
-1/4 C Almond Flour- 2 TBLS Coconut Flour
- 1/4 tsp Baking Powder -1 Egg
-add 1 tsp of your favorite seasoning
- Mix all together-
-Place in a mug (no need to grease).
-Microwave for 90 seconds!

For larger portion & oven!
-1/2 C Almond Flour -2 TBLS Coconut Flour
-1/2tsp Baking Powder -2 Eggs
-1 TBLS oil -1 TBLS water (if feels too thick)
-add salt & favorite seasoning
- Mix all together
-Place in a lined or greased small loaf pan
- Bake 20 min @ 350
*Note if you want larger loaf, double or triple the recipes
for thicker bread

Naturally GF
Low Glycemic Rolls

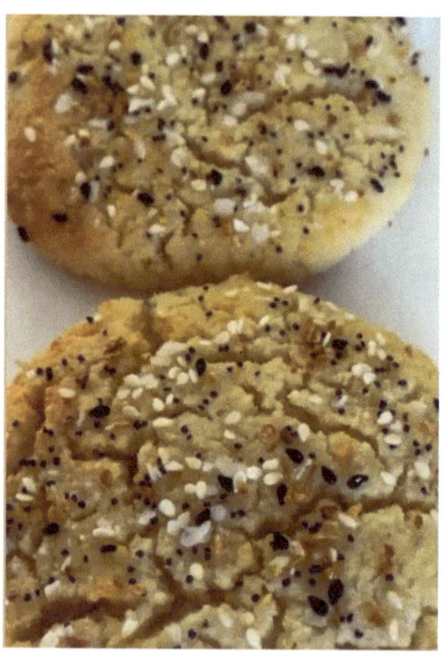

<u>5-INGREDIENTS</u>

-2 cups almond flour or oat flour (I used almond flour and they tasted like a biscuit!!)
-4 teaspoons baking powder -1 teaspoons kosher salt -2 cups plain Greek yogurt
-Everything bagel seasoning (or your favorite seasonings, cinnamon & coconut sugar or sesame seeds, dried onion flakes, dried garlic flakes, poppy seeds, etc. Be creative!)

<u>Directions-</u>

1. Preheat oven to 375 degrees F. Place parchment paper on a baking sheet.
2. In a bowl, mix together flour, baking powder and salt. Add the yogurt and mix until combined.
Mixture will be sticky.
3. Dust work surface with flour and place dough on top of floured surface. Knead the dough about 15 times until dough is combined and set aside some flour to sprinkle on top to flatten after placed on pan.
4. Divide into 8 balls. Roll each ball or your desired shape (bagel, roll, bun, round...) about 3/4- 1 inch thick.
5. Brush bagels with beaten egg whites (optional) and sprinkle with seasoning (a must for flavor).
6. Bake for 22 minutes on the top rack of the oven leaving space between bagels as they expand a little (if you use regular flour or any gluten flour they expand a lot more).
7. Enjoy!

*Stores on counter for 1 day and fridge for 3 days or can be frozen and then reheated.

3 Bonus Recipes

**Homemade Smoothie
By Rose's Wellness**

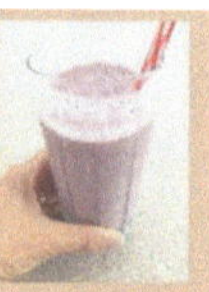

* * * * * * * * * * * * * * * * * *

1/2 or 1 C frozen berries
1/2 or 1 banana
1/2 or 1 C greek yogurt
2-4 TBSP ground flax
Water or Uns. Almond Milk
7-10 Sprinkles of Cinnamon

Rose's Wellness Immune Booster

STEP 1- Puree together
-Fresh squeezed lemon juice
(3 lg lemons)
-2 garlic cloves
-4, 1 inch peeled ginger pieces
-2 tsp turmeric
-2 tbls raw honey
STEP 2- Press pureer through
strainer into a large pitcher
STEP 3- add filtered or spring water

Ginger& Lemon Immune Booster

-Peel a 4 inch ginger and cut it in to 1 inch pieces
-squeeze the juice of 3 lemons
-place ginger & lemon juice in a blender & blend until pureed
-add 1 liter of filtered water to mixture
-blend water and the ginger/lemon all together
- strain the entire mixture into a pitcher & add ice
-throw the lemons in the pitcher for extra flavor
-add monk fruit or agave for extra sweetness
You can heat this up too!

The whole family will love these!

Bonus- Gluten Free Food List

Focus majority of diet on whole, nutrient dense, naturally gluten free foods.

Fruits, veggies, plant based proteins: beans, nuts, seeds, leant protein: chicken and fish.
Gluten Free whole grains, certified GF oats, brown or wild rice, quinoa, millet, amaranth, buckwheat, corn, sorghum & teff.
Nut flours (almond, oat, coconut). Bean flour (chickpea, red lentil, green lentil...)

What are you going to add to your grocery list?

____

____

____

____

____

____

____

____

____

____

____

Rose's Wellness

Thank you for purchasing this Ebook!
Stay healthy!
Live the best version of yourself!

For more guidance in creating the Life, Body & Health you desire... please visit www.roseswellness.com or email me at solutions@roseswellness.com